C 2017 by Marcia Mawae

ISBN 978 – 0 – 9988080 – 0 – 0

Scripture quotations are taken from The Living Bible,
Paraphrased, Copyright 1971 by Tyndale House Publishers, Inc., Carol Stream, Illinois 60188. All rights Reserved.

Library of Congress Cataloging-in-Publication Data
Mawae, Marcia Elliott
The Little Book of Dental Questions (for scaredycats and others)

Cover and Interior Pages by Andrew Myers

Self-published with CIP Block.com (P – CIP)

Printed in the United States of America

DEDICATION

To my family, especially my mom, who has always
supported and guided me. Also to Nicole, Marta, and
Lynne. And to my husband Kelii, who has always shown
me love and respect.

DISCLAIMER

Although the author and publisher have made every effort to ensure the information in this book was correct at print time, the aforementioned persons do not assume, and hereby disclaim, any liability to any party for any loss, damage, or disruption caused by errors or omissions, whether such errors or omissions result from negligence, accident, or any other cause.

The information in this book comes from the author's experience as a clinical dental hygienist, and as such is subjective -- i.e., the author's opinion. When in doubt with any questions regarding your teeth or mouth, you should consult with your dental hygienist or dentist for more information and clarification. All scripture quotations are taken from the Holy Bible.

"Get all the advice you can and be wise the rest of your life."

PROVERBS 19:20

TABLE OF CONTENTS

INTRODUCTION

Being a practicing dental hygienist for more than half my life has taught me many things. There are two kinds of patients: those who love going to the dentist, and those who don't. Neither group can relate easily to the other. And if you are one of those people in the first group, this book may not necessarily be for you! But I'll bet you know someone who might be in that second category, a brother or a friend. And the information might reinforce what you already know.

There are two ideas that have guided me throughout my life:

1.) My Christian upbringing has taught me I must treat others like I want to be treated.

2.) Ignorance is not bliss -- knowledge is bliss.

When we are in dental hygiene school, we start by working on mannequins instead of real people. When we get into the real world, we encounter real live patients who often have real fears, possibly even phobias, about going to the dentist! When a patient comes into my room, his/her body language often shows me that fear. But as I work with them, I love seeing this change, so when that person gets up to leave (when the appointment is finished), there is a smile on her face. And I have found that the way to that end result is through two things: knowledge and comfort. Trust will come and is most important; e.g., if a person understands me and is comfortable, then we are both happy. That person can relax and trust me, and then I can do my job more easily. So that is the purpose of this little book. I hope to answer some of the questions everyone has -- the questions people have been asking me for many years; there is much misinformation out there; I would like to clear this up, to share what I have learned. Then, hopefully, your experience going to the dentist can be a happy one.

We hygienists treat the whole person, knowing that our health in general is affected by a healthy mouth. Our mouths being the dirtiest part of our bodies bacteria-wise, it follows that if we have infection in our mouths, it can affect our health as well as our very lives!

I also thank all my great patients: I have learned as much from them as I hope they have learned from me. I have been blessed to be able to help many people. They have left the office feeling better from what I have done, and that, more than any fee, has made my work worthwhile.

"God comforts us so that we comfort those in any trouble."

2 CORINTHIANS 1:4

How do I find a good dentist/dental hygienist that's right for me?

You can ask your friends, family members, or co-workers. Choose someone, though, who has the same standards as yours for dental care. We all have different priorities, whether it be cost, comfort, aesthetics, or others. And you need to be able to communicate comfortably with your dental professional. You can also look online using the same standards. The professional needs to be sensitive to your needs and to be able to listen, as well as have good communication skills that you understand.

If you're not happy with your choice, have the confidence to get a second opinion; keep looking until you find someone you are happy with.

"Ask where the good way is, and walk in it, and you will find rest for your souls."

JEREMIAH 6:16

Why am I so afraid to go to the dentist?

There are three main reasons why people do not go to the dentist:

1. FINANCES

Dentistry can be expensive, especially if you don't have dental insurance. But think of it this way: The longer you wait to see a dentist, the more expensive it will get, as little problems become big problems! Prevention is always better.

2. IGNORANCE

Many people have not been told by their parents or others how important it is to take care of their teeth. Regardless of level of education or financial station, they believe what their parents taught (or did not teach) them.

3. FEAR

This is a huge factor. Some fear comes from past experience, or even hearing scary stories from a friend or family member. There are centers throughout the country that deal very effectively with dental "phobics." Aromatherapy (e.g., lavender oil), hypnosis, acupressure, a mild sedative, and massage can help.

"My Christian experience tells me that God has not given us a spirit of fear, But of power and love"

2 TIMOTHY 1:7, PARAPHRASED

What is the difference between a dental hygienist and a dental assistant?

The word "dental," in Latin, refers to teeth. Dentists have trained dental assistants to help them with their patients in the office. Dental assistants can be formally trained in school, or they can be trained in the office by the dentist. Dental hygienists, on the other hand, work independently from the dentist in the office. They are formally trained in two to four years, often receiving a college degree if they attend a four-year school. "Hygiene," in Latin, means "clean." So dental hygienists, among other responsibilities, clean your teeth and are educated in many ways, similar to a nurse, to help prevent disease in your mouth. Therefore, one of a hygienist's primary jobs is educating our patients. Our methods for doing this are also self-serving: If we can give our patients the knowledge they need about how to care for their mouths, it also makes our job easier!

My Christian faith tells me that our bodies are His temple, that we must take care of the body...very important.

"Can't you hear the voice of wisdom? She is standing at the city gates and at every fork in the road, and at the door of every house. Listen to what she says."

PROVERBS 8:1-3

When I go to the dentist, I am so distracted that I often forget what my dentist or hygienist is telling me after I leave the office!

According to a study done in 2003 by Sherpa Research Centre, 40–80% of the information provided by healthcare professionals is immediately forgotten by the patient, and almost half the information patients do remember is incorrect! A stressful situation can cause this to happen -- patients are not always focused listeners. And dental professionals often use "dental jargon" that people don't understand. **Solutions include:**

1. Repeating the information we are given solidifies it in our brain.

2. Writing down the information also helps: Either the patient or the dental professional can do this

3. Asking questions is also a good idea. Again, either the patient or the dental professional can do this.

"I have learned the secret of being content...
whether living in plenty or in want. I can do everything
through Him who gives me strength."

PHILIPPIANS 4:12-13

What is the difference between plaque and tartar?

People very often get confused about the difference between plaque (biofilm) and tartar (calculus). It is actually pretty simple, if you think about it:

Plaque is soft, and this pasty film forms every day, coming from the bacteria in your mouth. If you can picture the plaque that forms in your blood vessels, the plaque in your mouth can be pictured the same way. Plaque is the matrix that bacteria create and live in. It is easily removed when we correctly brush and floss.

Tartar, on the other hand, is hard and cannot be removed with a toothbrush and floss. Tartar is a mineral deposit, calcium, that comes from our saliva. Because it is hard and feels rough to our tongue, it can irritate and eventually start infection (along with bacteria) in the gum tissue. Tartar needs to be professionally removed by a dental hygienist or dentist.

"A person's wisdom yields patience..."

PROVERBS 19:10

Why do I get so much tartar when I feel I do a good job brushing and flossing?

Because tartar forms independently from plaque, there are ways we can control it more effectively:

1. Tartar control toothpastes and mouth rinses help, in part by chemically binding with the calcium deposits (tartar) before they attach to our teeth.

2. Smoking can dry the plaque and tartar faster, and stain from smoking can make a rough surface on the teeth that helps the tartar to attach. If you smoke, quit smoking!

3. Allergies that cause us to breathe through our mouths more can also cause plaque and tartar to dry faster. Mouth breathers quite often have gum tissue inflammation too, since the moisture in our mouths is one way we are protected from the bacteria. Brushing your teeth more often helps, and you can also get your teeth cleaned more frequently (every 3-4 months instead of every 6 months).

4. Heredity can also be a factor: Just as we inherit the color of our eyes, we also inherit our tendency to form tartar. And some people believe that if you have more high-calcium foods in your diet, this can contribute to tartar buildup. Again, more frequent dental cleanings helps.

If you have been told by your dental professional that you are a tartar-former (Some people get mostly plaque, not tartar), concentrate on cleaning your lower front teeth and your upper molars. Because the tartar-forming calcium comes from your salivary glands, know that your primary glands are around these teeth.

"My dear brothers and sisters, take note of this: Everyone should be quick to listen, slow to speak..."

JAMES 1:19

Why do I have to brush and floss every day?

Aside from the fact that our teeth feel better when they are shiny and clean and we can smile with confidence, we might not realize that it takes about 24 hours for us to build up a layer of plaque (biofilm). That is what kids say makes our teeth feel "fuzzy." The process of cleaning our teeth helps to disorganize the bacterial colonies that cause plaque to form. So we are basically killing the bacteria that cause gum disease and cavities as well as bad breath.

We are also helping to prevent stains and tartar (calculus) from forming, as well as cleaning out particles.

"A merry heart doeth good like medicine;
but a broken spirit drieth the bones."

PROVERBS 17:22

What's the best way to brush my teeth?

Good question! If you are using a recommended soft or extra-soft toothbrush, make sure you angle it at about 45 degrees into the gum area on your teeth. A back-and-forth "sawing" motion can wear down your enamel, so a circular motion is best; or you can use a short side-to-side motion. It's also not good to brush up and down on your front teeth, as this tends to push your gum tissue down and may also push the plaque under your gums. If your teeth are sensitive, using a rolling motion can help.

If you are using an electric toothbrush, make sure you don't use a brushing motion -- just hold the brush at the same recommended angle and keep the brush steady for five seconds, then move on to the next area and repeat. The brushing motion you would use with a hand brush can cancel out the benefits of the high-speed vibration and is not really necessary. Some people are more sensitive to the electric brush's vibration, and they tell me that using their brush later in the day seems to help to prevent this.

And don't forget to brush the chewing surface plus your tongue (gently), the roof of your mouth, and the inside of your cheeks. The area most people tend to miss when brushing is at the gumline -- pay extra attention to this area, remembering to brush your gums as well. People who have longer teeth need to brush twice: once at the gumline and a second time at the edges of their teeth. If you've ever heard the expression that a person is "long in the tooth," this mostly comes with age, as our gums naturally recede. (I once had a patient who told me everything was receding -- his hairline, waistline, and gumline!) By the way, the correct amount of time to brush your teeth is actually two full minutes...and electric brushes are already timed to stay on for this length of time.

> "My Christian faith tells me, "Don't you realize that your body is the temple of the Holy Spirit?"

1 CORINTHIANS 6:19

What is the best toothbrush for me?

Toothbrushes come in all sizes, kinds, and textures. You should choose one that fits comfortably in your hand and its bristles reach easily around the backside of your last molar. There are toothbrushes so large that they look more like a shoe brush, with the idea that they will cover a larger area effectively. However, a smaller toothbrush seems to work better to get around corners and small areas. Although some people say they prefer a firm or hard bristle toothbrush, these are dangerous because, combined with more abrasive toothpaste, they can actually wear away your enamel, causing sensitivity and possible decay as you wear into the softer dentin underneath your tooth's enamel. In addition, a stiffer toothbrush ends up just swiping across the tooth surface, rather than getting around the curves of the teeth. By the way, if you see deep grooves starting to appear, especially on the front side of your teeth at the gumline, this could be the previously mentioned toothbrush wear.

Electric toothbrushes are popular and are actually more effective: The approximately 31,000 vibrations per minute of an adult electric brush do a better job of cleaning your teeth, strengthening your gums, and breaking up bacterial colonies (therefore killing bacteria). Electric toothbrushes are actually less abrasive than hand toothbrushes!

"But you, be strong and do not let your hands be weak,
for your work shall be rewarded."

2 CHRONICLES 15:7

How can I keep my toothbrush cleaner?

1. Remember: It's important to replace your toothbrush every three months, whether it is an electric (not the handle) or hand brush, for two reasons: It collects bacteria, and the bristles can get too soft, so that they bend and miss the sulcus area (the area where the tooth and the gum meet) and don't clean effectively.

2. If you have a cold or some other communicable disease, it is important to replace your toothbrush right away.

3. Some people like to place their brush (not electric!) in the dishwasher.

4. You can dip your brush in an antibacterial mouthwash.

5. Never put your toothbrush in the medicine cabinet or any other enclosed area: A cool dark place is a perfect breeding ground for bacteria.

6. Close your toilet lid. When you flush the toilet the bacteria in it can travel out about 10 feet, which is important if your toothbrush is within this range.

"Let the favor of the Lord our God be upon us. And make the work of our hands Stand strong. Yes, make the work of our hands stand strong."

PSALMS 90:17

Why do I need to floss?

You can brush your teeth forever, and yet your toothbrush will never clean completely between your teeth. We floss for the same reason we brush: to clean out food, to help prevent stain and plaque formation, and, most importantly, to disorganize (kill) bacteria in the plaque that causes cavities, bad breath, and gum infection. Remember: The more you do on a daily basis, the less we have to do when you visit the dental office. And that is the best plan for preventive dentistry. This way, everyone's happy, since you are more comfortable and we don't have to work so hard!

There is a correct way to floss: Move back and forth with the floss to get past the tight contacts between the teeth. Then, move the floss up and down to cover the whole side of the tooth, making sure you go into the space under your gum (sulcus). Don't forget to floss the back side of the last tooth in each corner. Try to curve the floss around your tooth, which is curved itself; you'll cover more area that way. It's good to floss at least 1-2 times a day. Use about 1-½ to 2 feet of floss. Wrap the floss around the middle finger of each hand; then, use your thumbs and forefingers to control the floss. Wrap it on/off your fingers as you go along; that way you will have a clean area of floss in between each two teeth.

**"Listen to advice and accept discipline,
and at the end you will be counted among the wise."**

PROVERBS 19:20

What is the best floss to use, and what if I cannot floss?

The best floss for you is the one you like and will use! There are all kinds: waxed, unwaxed, tape, extra fine, woven, and Teflon-coated, to name a few. Extra fine, woven, or waxed flosses work well if your teeth are very close together (tight contacts). If you can get the floss in but it breaks when you try to pull it back out, you can try pulling the floss out sideways. There are also slingshot-shaped pre-threaded flossers for people who have dexterity problems; these work well for kids too. You can also buy all sorts of small picks and brushes, for use in-between your teeth.

Another option, though it might not take the place of the above-mentioned devices for the scraping action, is a water irrigator. These are very easy to use, and do a good job killing bacteria as well as strengthening your gums. They can also go deeper if you have gum recession underneath (pockets). Make sure you start with the lowest water pressure and gradually increase it: Although it feels good to hike the pressure up high in the beginning, this is actually too forceful and can damage the gum tissue. If you choose to add other ingredients in addition to water in the receptacle, be sure to flush through the lines with plain water afterward, to keep your appliance from getting clogged. It really is not necessary to add anything, since the pulsing of the water alone is what breaks up the bacterial colonies.

"A person's wisdom yields patience..."

PROVERBS 19:11

14

I just bought a water irrigator that was recommended by my dental hygienist -- is this safe to use in my mouth?

Water irrigators are very popular now. There are two kinds, and they both work well. The original "tub" version has actually been around for many years. It lost popularity, primarily because people were using it incorrectly and it was causing damage to the gum tissue. It's become popular again, with the understanding that certain careful instructions must be adhered to. The second type of irrigator is a handheld device similar in size to an electric toothbrush. With this type, you fill a compartment in the handle with water.

The most important instruction you must remember is to start out with your irrigator on the very lowest pressure. It's effective at this level even though you might not feel like it is. Then, you can gradually turn up the pressure over a few days' time. Using the highest pressure in the beginning is too forceful and can actually do damage and seriously irritate your gum tissue.

Some people like to add different antibacterial or healing liquids to the water receptacle. Be careful if you do this because it can eventually clog the appliance. And there's really no need to add anything else, since the way the water pulses out is what's killing bacteria, breaking up the bacterial colonies. But if you prefer to add other liquids, make sure you flush through the lines with plain water when you are finished using it. Another alternative is to just rinse with your favorite liquid from a glass after you are finished with the irrigator.

Irrigators are great for strengthening (massaging) your gums, and also for getting into deeper pockets and hard-to-reach areas. This will, of course, keep your mouth healthier. Irrigators alone may not give you the scraping action of floss, so ideally you should use both.

"May you have loving favor and peace from God our Father."

EPHESIANS 1:3

I get confused about which toothpaste is the best one for me...

Your dental professional can help you with this. Remember that "one size does not fit all"...In other words, the best toothpaste for you might not be best for other members of your family.

1. Tartar control toothpastes are best for those who accumulate tartar. There are various amounts of this ingredient in different toothpastes; the cheaper toothpastes might not be as effective.

2. Antibacterial toothpastes: These help prevent cavities, bad breath, plaque formation, and gum infection.

3. Enamel-building toothpastes: These are good if your enamel is thin, if you are more prone to cavity formation, or if your teeth are sensitive.

4. Whitening toothpastes: There are two kinds:

    *   Abrasive toothpastes, which can help remove or prevent stain, but will not change the actual shade of your teeth. Be careful with these because they can gradually wear away your enamel, causing possible sensitivity!
    *   Actual whitening toothpastes that may change the shade of your enamel, but with minimal real effect.

NOTE: It is always good to make sure your toothpaste or rinse has the ADA stamp of approval on the package. This indicates the item has been tested and approved for safe use.

"...Whatever is true...think on these things."

PHILIPPIANS 4:8

What about "natural" dental products?

Many people prefer natural toothpastes, rinses, and other natural products. Before using any of these, though, it's important that you get reliable information from a dental professional about the product's safety. Both green and black teas may work like natural decay-preventatives; black tea is five times more effective for this. Tea tree oil from a particular kind of tea tree has antibacterial as well as antifungal properties.

Baking soda, which has a basic pH (the opposite of acidic), can help counteract the acidity in your mouth so that it is able to kill bacteria, which thrive in an acidic environment. It also helps to control the cold sore virus and limits staining but is less abrasive than a lot of toothpastes. I like straight baking soda for brushing; one teaspoon in about a half-cup of warm water is good for a rinse.

There are several natural products you can get online or in health food stores...just make sure you check with a professional before using them!

"Wisdom is a tree of life to those who eat her fruit;
happy is the man who keeps eating it."

PROVERBS 3:18

I saw a commercial advertising on TV about a dental product... How do I know if it's safe?

Remember, advertisers can make all kinds of claims about their product. Also, remember that a major motivation for this is for their profit. The advertised product may or may not be OK to use. The American Dental Association (ADA) has its own standards of safety for dental products; look for the ADA stamp of approval that indicates the product has been tested for safety. You can also consult your dentist or hygienist: They are up to date on products based on their required continuing education courses and from printed literature.

"Be at peace with all men."

HEBREWS 12:14

What about mouth rinses?

There are two basic uses for rinses: prevention and treatment.

1. For healing purposes, warm salt water rinses are good. And for people who get cold sores inside or outside their mouths, baking soda rinses are helpful, although these sores must heal on their own -- the baking soda just makes the sores less uncomfortable while healing. For both of these, you can add one teaspoonful to about half a cup of warm water. Some people like to use hydrogen peroxide diluted half-and-half with warm water. Antibacterial rinses help control cavity-causing bacteria as well as those that cause bad breath and gum infection.

2. Fluoride rinses, used after brushing and flossing, can help keep your enamel hard.

3. Antiplaque and tartar-control rinses help keep your teeth cleaner.

Try to make sure you use a rinse that has no alcohol, as this can irritate and dry your mouth. If you do have an alcohol-containing rinse, it's good to dilute it half-and-half with water. The best time to rinse is after, not before, you brush and floss. And try not to eat or drink for about 30 minutes after rinsing, to get more benefits.

"He shall be like a tree planted by the rivers of water, that brings forth its fruit in season. Whose leaf also shall not wither; and whatever he does shall prosper."

PSALMS 1:3

I am physically challenged with a disability that affects my hands. Can you recommend any good items for me to clean my teeth?

There are many good products for sale for anyone with disabilities or handicaps. A Y-shaped floss aid that looks like a slingshot can be used with one hand. A water irrigator is also very effective and easy to use. Nursing homes, hospitals, and medical supply stores can provide a cleaner shaped like a small foam piece with a lollipop-type handle. Electric toothbrushes are helpful and basically do the work for you, and are more effective than a handheld toothbrush. Rinsing can also be helpful -- both healing rinses such as salt water, and preventive rinses such as fluoride, anti-plaque, and tartar control.

**"I know that you can do all things.
Nothing can put a stop to your plans."**

JOB 42:2

Why do I have to get my teeth cleaned?

My husband always asks me this question. He brushes his teeth regularly, he says, and he thinks that should be enough. I respond to him that if brushing alone were that effective, we wouldn't need dental hygienists! We hygienists have very good job security for this reason, especially since our bodies form tartar (calculus), even when we brush and floss daily. When hygienists clean your teeth (prophylaxis or prophy) we are looking for five things: food, plaque, tartar, stain, and bacteria. As with so many things, the culprit we cannot see is what causes the most damage: bacteria. So, the most important item for you to remove daily through brushing, flossing, and many other home tools, is bacteria. Plaque also is created by bacteria, and it takes only about 24 hours to accumulate a layer of plaque (biofilm).

"Beloved, I wish above all things that thou mayest prosper and be in good health, even as thy soul prospereth.

3 JOHN 1:2

What can I do to help prevent cavities?

Remember, there are lots of "hidden" sugars as well as acidy drinks. The sugar we put in our coffee or tea, particularly honey, is an example. And most sports drinks contain much more acid than soda. Not to mention fruit juices, lemon in our glass of water, etc. Prevention is the key word here. What you put into your mouth, combined with decay-causing bacteria, is what causes a cavity to form. Your enamel is the hardest surface in your body, even harder than your bones. But certain bacteria (different from the bacteria that cause gum disease) can break down any carbohydrate in your mouth, especially simple carbohydrates like sugar. The resulting by-product of this action is acid. Because our enamel is so hard, there are only a few things that can damage it. Enamel is only vulnerable to cracks, chips, and acid. There are other kinds of acid such as vinegar. Incidentally, some people just naturally inherit thinner enamel. Also, people with eating disorders like bulimia can produce stomach acid in their mouths, which can dissolve the enamel. So, any food or drink we ingest that has sugar or acid should be avoided.

Of course, we all like sweets, so there are several things we can do to halt this acid production. It takes about 20 minutes for our mouth's bacteria to break down sugar and start producing acid. What can we do in that 20-minute time frame to help?

1. The ideal solution is to brush and floss. But we are in many situations where this is not convenient, so:

2. Rinsing your mouth with water or a mouthwash immediately after ingesting acidic liquids or sugar dilutes the acid.

3. Certain mouthwashes contain an antibacterial ingredient to kill the bacteria.

4. Chewing sugarless gum can help produce saliva that also dilutes the acid. Some people believe that Xylitol gum helps.

5. Fluoride rinses help keep the enamel stronger.

6. Enamel-building toothpastes can also help strengthen the enamel.

**"Do you like honey? Don't eat too much of it,
or it will make you sick!"**

PROVERBS 25:16

I drink a lot of sugar-free drinks -- is this OK?

Sugar-free drinks are OK in moderation, but you also need to remember that even these drinks contain certain acids that can damage your enamel. Drinks that are very high in acids -- higher than soda -- are the popular sports drinks. Also, don't forget that putting lemon or lime juice in your drinking water can be damaging. If you choose to drink these beverages, it's best to make it a habit to rinse your mouth with plain water as a follow-up. Of course, plain drinking water is actually the healthiest for our teeth as well as our bodies.

"Sing and make music from your heart to the Lord,
always giving thanks to God the Father for everything."

EPHESIANS 5:19-20

How can I tell whether my tongue is healthy?

Sometimes we get a coating on our tongue, which can be an indication of a low-grade infection, either bacterial or yeast in origin. Our tongue can sometimes feel sore too. Certain foods, such as milk, can create a coating. And remember to clean your tongue regularly but gently. You can use your toothbrush or a tongue scraper.

Did you know your tongue is the strongest muscle in your body relative to size? It helps us to talk, eat, swallow, taste, and clean our teeth. We have different taste buds on our tongue to help us differentiate between foods that are sweet, salty, bitter, or sour. Eating disorders like bulimia can cause damage to the taste buds, so people with this disorder prefer spicier foods because they cannot taste flavors as well. And don't forget that your taste comes from your nose's sense of smell.

Some people pierce their tongues, a popular trend: If you decide to do this, make sure you use a licensed professional. And plastic ornaments are much safer than metal, which can chip your teeth.

In general, it's always best to seek professional help if you have any questions or concerns.

"The tongue of the wise brings healing."

PROVERBS 12:18

I worry sometimes that I have bad, offensive breath. What causes this and how can I prevent it?

There are several causes of bad breath that can come from other areas of your body. If you have a problem with excess stomach acid, this can cause malodor. Sinus infections (sinusitis) that produce drainage of the infected fluid down the back of your throat can be another cause. And people who have uncontrolled diabetes can have fetid breath. Another very common cause can be either gum disease or an abscessed or decayed tooth.

For garlic or other temporary malodors, a tongue scraper and/or mouth rinses can help; approximately 80 percent of odor-causing bacteria reside on your tongue. If the problem persists, it's best to seek medical and dental professional help.

"...And with your wisdom, develop common sense and good judgment... listen to me and do as I say, and you will have a long, good life."

PROVERBS 4:7

How can I prevent bad breath?

Bad breath can be caused by many different things, such as sinusitis, smoking, and indigestion. Some causes require medical advice. And a decayed or infected tooth can cause a bad odor. Another major cause of bad breath is gum disease: This requires screening and treatment by your dentist or dental hygienist. After a detailed gum exam is performed, usually accompanied by x-rays, the treatment will normally require anywhere from one to four dental cleanings where local anesthetic is typically administered. In advanced stages of gum disease where your teeth have loosened from bone loss, it might even require tooth extractions. Sometimes a referral to a gum specialist (periodontist) is advised. Regular dental cleanings can often prevent this malady.

Brushing the top surface of the tongue or using a specially made tongue scraper daily can also help, as up to 80 percent of the bacteria that cause bad breath reside on your tongue. Rinses can also help, but choose one that has little or no alcohol, as the alcohol can have a tendency to burn your mouth. The antibacterial ingredients are what you're looking for. Also, it is a good idea to wait 30 minutes after rinsing before eating, so the rinse has a longer time to effectively kill the bacteria that cause bad breath. Of course, it's understood that common culprits such as garlic and onions are also responsible for unpleasant breath!

"...Take note of this: Everyone should be quick to listen."

JAMES 1:19

Why do I need x-rays at the dentist?
I'm nervous about too much radiation.

Radiation is an important tool, not only for medical and dental diagnosis, but also for treatment in cancer patients as well as other cases: One example for its use is to help prevent excessive scar tissue on the skin (keloids).

In dentistry, "x-rays," or radiographs, help us to find problems such as decay, bone loss, and any suspicious lesions. Since we don't have "x-ray vision," it's the best way to see what's going on inside the tissue, often preventing bigger problems. Of course, we do need to be careful with its use, and there is new technology that provides much safer radiation dosage; e.g., the high-speed film that dental offices use now. Digital radiographs are the latest development and allow much less radiation exposure. And it's interesting to note that people who usually are exposed to the most radiation have traditionally been airplane pilots: They are closer to the original radiation source: the sun!

"Timely advice is as lovely as golden apples in a silver basket."

PROVERBS 25:11

My friend told me his dental office takes digital x-rays...

Digital x-rays (radiographs) are a very popular trend in dentistry, and they involve a computer. One nice advantage is that they require much less radiation than traditional film x-rays, which is healthier for the patient. Another new device in dentistry is the laser. Lasers can be used to remove unhealthy tissue in the mouth: Periodontists and oral surgeons often use a laser to perform this procedure. And some lasers can actually regenerate bone in the mouth for patients with severe bone loss. Using a laser is cleaner because it can also kill harmful bacteria. Lasers can be used by a general dentist, hygienist, or other dental specialists.

A panoramic radiograph can show the entire mouth on one large film, helping to show issues such as generalized bone loss and lesions in the mouth. Individual radiographs (periapical and bitewing films) are good for displaying more detail or definition, but cannot show the whole picture.

Camera wands or intraoral cameras can also be used for diagnosis. These cameras, a little larger than an ink pen, are a takeoff on endoscopes used in the medical profession. Because they generally magnify about 30 times, it is possible to find such things as cracks in teeth and fillings breaking down much earlier.

"Jesus said to her, 'Daughter, your faith has healed you.
Go in peace and be free from your suffering.' "

MARK 5:34

What is this brown spot on my tooth?

I can understand why this can be very alarming, partly because we in the dental profession have trained everyone to worry that this spot might be a cavity. Tooth staining can come from any dark-colored food or drink we ingest: juice, tea, or coffee. And one of the worst causes is smoking. Stain can settle on the tooth surface or into a white filling or tooth: "intrinsic" stain. Some toothpastes are more abrasive and can control surface stain. (Be careful with more abrasive toothpastes, as they can wear away the tooth enamel and often cause tooth sensitivity!) It often helps to brush with baking soda, which is less abrasive. Rinsing after drinking stain-causing liquids can help prevent staining. And drinking your coffee or tea without cream or milk helps prevent staining, as the cream/milk leaves a film on the teeth that can make it easier for the stain to attach.

Tooth brushing also helps prevent staining; electric toothbrushes are more effective at this. But the only true way to know if a stain is a cavity is, of course, to see your dental professional.

"Anxious hearts are heavy but a word
of encouragement does wonders."

PROVERBS 12:25

My gum tissue looks funny to me --
do I need to have this checked?

Dental textbooks traditionally describe healthy gum tissue as "coral pink," and unhealthy tissue is usually a bright red color. The textbook shade usually refers to a Caucasian person, but there can be variations of this color that are quite normal, as some dark-skinned cultures naturally can have darker or even black-pigmented gum tissue. Very hot foods and drinks or spicy foods can irritate your mouth. And smoking, of course, is a major irritant; long-time smokers' gum tissue can sometimes look gray, as the heat/nicotine irritants cause the gums to build up a tough fibrous layer. An oral exam should be included as part of a regular dental visit. It's best to see your dentist or dental hygienist to make sure everything in your mouth is healthy.

"Kind words are like honey -- enjoyable and healthful."

PROVERBS 16:24

Why are my teeth so yellow?

Different factors can cause your teeth to look yellow. People who have inherited thicker enamel can have teeth that appear less white. But one advantage to this is that they are less likely to get cavities. Food and drinks that are a darker color, as well as smoking, can darken your teeth. Your enamel is actually porous, like a sponge, so over time it will absorb the stain. But sometimes the stain is only on the surface, and if you can get your teeth cleaned it can help remove the stain. Poor oral hygiene can also contribute. As we get older, our teeth will generally become more yellow. (Our teeth normally start out with a creamy color.) Dark-skinned people, as well as women's darker lipstick shades, can give the appearance, by contrast, of whiter teeth. And avoiding white clothing around your face can help your teeth appear whiter. Electric toothbrushes can help prevent staining. Brushing with baking soda or a "whitening " toothpaste can help prevent staining as well. Another popular solution is to cosmetically whiten your teeth.

"Peace I leave you; my peace I give you. I do not give you as the world gives. Do not let your hearts be troubled and do not be afraid."

JOHN 14:27

What is periodontal disease and how can I prevent it?

Periodontal or gum disease is the biggest cause of tooth loss, partly because its symptoms are often painless. This can unfortunately lead people to think they have no problems, even though there are signs such as bad breath and bleeding gums. Smoking, which is a major cause of gum disease, can trick you into a false sense of security because the cigarette's heat and nicotine cause the gum tissue to form a tough fibrous layer of protection. Meanwhile, the infection is still progressing out of sight, under your gums. Quit smoking!! By the way, marijuana and clove cigarettes can also be a danger.

Certain medications can also contribute to gum disease. Stress is another huge factor, as our mind and emotions can affect our bodies right down to the cellular level. And we now understand that there is a connection between many health problems, such as heart and lung disease, and gum infection.

Getting your teeth cleaned and checked regularly is the best way to help prevent this problem, because tartar and plaque buildup, along with bacteria, are the main contributing factors. If not checked, this buildup can start the gum infection; then, the gums and bone begin to recede underneath, where we cannot see the infection happening. Eventually the teeth become loose due to lack of gum and bone support. Bacteria-wise, our mouth is the dirtiest part of our body. So regular dental visits are not only important to make our teeth look good, but they can actually help us save our teeth as well as save our lives!

"Timely advice is as lovely as golden apples in a silver basket."

PROVERBS 25:1

Why are my teeth so sensitive?

Did you know you have more nerves in your head than anywhere else in your body?! This naturally makes your mouth more sensitive. According to research, by the way, men have a lower tolerance for pain in general -- a lower pain threshold -- than women. And some people are just naturally more sensitive: They'll be more apt to jump if someone comes up behind them, or if they hear a loud noise. These people tend to have more sensitive teeth and gum tissue. Brushing incorrectly can cause sensitivity; electric toothbrushes in general are less apt to contribute to this. Different whitening products and toothpastes can make your teeth more sensitive too, so switching to a less abrasive toothpaste or one made for enamel building/desensitizing can help. If you choose the latter, try not to rinse or put anything in your mouth for a few minutes after you brush; otherwise, you can remove the desensitizing ingredient before it has a chance to work. A cavity will usually cause sensitivity, and you will need to see a dental professional if your teeth become sensitive to hot.

"Have two goals: wisdom...and common sense.
Don't let them slip away"

PROVERBS 3:21

My mouth often feels too dry -- is this normal?

If you are a mouth-breather (allergies can cause you to breathe through your mouth if your nose is stopped up), your mouth can be over-dry. Also, there are over 300 medications that can dry your mouth. And as we get older, with midlife our salivary glands change and can produce less saliva. Anyone who has undergone radiation treatments in an area close to the mouth can have a dry mouth, as the salivary glands are affected by this. A condition called Sjogren's Syndrome can also cause the mouth to dry out, as this health problem can affect many glands in the body.

A dry mouth can be dangerous, as moisture in your mouth is a key way the mouth is protected against bacteria that cause gum disease as well as tooth decay. Check with your dental professional or pharmacist about rinses and gels that can protect your mouth, including fluoride rinses. Chewing sugarless gum can help produce more saliva. Drinking lots of water throughout the day is important, as well as brushing and flossing more often.

"...if you pay attention to His commands and keep all His decrees, I will not bring on you any of the diseases."

EXODUS 15:26

I've noticed I am getting deep grooves on the front of my teeth at my gumline. Is this normal?

Your teeth have a small indentation in them at the gumline, where the crown part of your tooth meets the root; this is normal. But if these grooves are getting deeper, this can be dangerous, as your dentin (the material underneath the enamel) becomes more exposed. One cause for this can be over-brushing, especially brushing incorrectly, or with a harder-bristled brush. More abrasive toothpastes can also contribute. If you use a long, "sawing"-type stroke, this can be corrected to a circular or roll-type technique, as well as switching to a softer toothbrush, which we actually recommend. A good choice of toothbrush is an electric brush that is much more thorough, but less abrasive.

Another cause can be "abfractions." This happens most often with people who grind or clench their teeth. With this "torquing," a wedge of your tooth can pop off. But it is very important to get this checked, as exposed dentin can cause sensitivity or even a cavity. A dental professional can advise you on this problem.

**"So lift up your hands that have been weak.
Stand up on your weak legs. Walk straight ahead so the weak
leg will not be turned aside, but will be healed."**

HEBREWS 12:12

When I chew, I sometimes hear a "clicking" noise in my jaw -- is this normal?

Your jaw connects to your skull by way of what we call a "temporomandibular joint (TMJ)." Just like when you hear or feel joints clicking anywhere else in your body, this clicking can, if left untreated, become painful as the muscles and ligaments surrounding this area get more irritated. See your dental professional, especially if it gets worse, to find possible solutions to this problem. Sometimes we do things that can temporarily cause irritation to this joint, like opening our mouths too wide, chewing gum, or eating very chewy foods. Taking a break from these behaviors, using ice packs, or taking over-the-counter painkiller anti-inflammatory medication can help. Sometimes there is a problem with your occlusion (bite). A bite adjustment can help, and in severe cases orthodontics might be recommended.

"...we also glory in our sufferings, because we know that suffering produces; perseverance, character; and character, hope."

ROMANS 5:3-4

My teeth seem to be wearing down on the chewing surface. What can I do to prevent this?

We all have different habits, some of which are not good and can affect our teeth. Nail-biting and chewing ice are major contributing factors to tooth wear, chipping, and cracking. Another important cause is bruxism (grinding) and the related clenching of our teeth. We know that these latter two habits can be strongly hereditary: A person can inherit this habit from their parent and then, in turn, pass it on to their child. The sound children make when grinding is very noticeable, as the child does this mostly during sleep. Adults also clench or grind during their sleep, which is harder for them to recognize. But this can manifest symptoms such as a sore jaw, shooting head pain, and headaches.

Stress or an overactive day can usually contribute to this habit. So, solutions for prevention can include exercise, yoga, massage, or anything to help you relax. A very good option is a device you can have made at your dental office called a mouthguard. This lightweight device is inserted at bedtime and covers most of the upper teeth, preventing tooth contact that causes grinding or clenching. Your dental professional can also check your occlusion (bite) to determine if it's not normal. And in some cases, orthodontics might be recommended.

"My brethren, count it all joy when you fall into various trials."

JAMES 1:2

I just found out I am pregnant. Is there any important information about my teeth I need to know?

Of course, you need to have good nutrition at this time -- even more important, since you are eating for two! "Morning sickness" can create a more acidic environment in your mouth, which is not good for your teeth. You might want to add a fluoride rinse to your daily regimen as a preventative. There is also a condition called "pregnancy gingivitis" that affects most women who are expecting; this is caused by the hormone changes in your body during pregnancy. It can cause your gums to swell and bleed more easily. Warm salt water rinses can help with this; and, of course, brushing and flossing more often is a good idea. You need to address this problem right away, because if you don't, the bacteria in your mouth can turn this into gum inflammation and ultimately infection...and it might not go away, even after you have your baby.

"...Be strong and of good courage -- do not be afraid..."

JOSHUA 1:7

I want to plan now, before I have my baby, to do the best for my child. Do you have advice you can give me about this?

First of all, if you decide to breastfeed, this can be a good thing for many reasons. Did you know that when you begin to breastfeed, the first ingredient you give your baby is actually natural antibiotics to help protect your baby from infection? And any time after the baby is born, it's very important that you do not put your baby to bed with a bottle containing milk or juice, even diluted. If these liquids puddle in the baby's mouth, it can be a problem. This dangerous habit, called "Baby Bottle Syndrome," is a major cause of cavities in young children. Teeth usually start to erupt around 6 months of age, and all 20 teeth normally come in around age 2, although you need not be alarmed if your baby's teeth come in earlier or later than this. After teething is finished, it's recommended that you take your child to the dentist for their first visit. Actually, the American Dental Association recommends a child's first dental visit at around age 1. An exception to this, of course, is if you see any suspicious spots, if your child has an accident loosening or knocking out teeth, etc. You may choose to take your child to either a general dentist or a pedodontist (children's dentist).

Some children can be a little afraid to come to the dentist, so for that reason, the first visit should be very short, so your child can gradually get more comfortable. Some offices allow you to come into the room with the child, or even let him or her sit on your lap in the chair. If you do this, make sure you show no signs of fear or nervousness yourself, as children readily pick up on this. The first visit should be a pleasant experience for everyone!

**"Open your heart to teaching,
and your ears to words of much learning."**

PSALM 23:12

I get cold sores often. How can I prevent this?

There does seem to be a general hereditary tendency for some people to get cold sores and canker sores. There are actually two different viruses that cause these: herpes simplex and herpes zoster. The first causes cold sores inside your mouth, and the second outside your mouth, although they can also appear in other areas of your body. Often, they can occur on the outside of your lips, and the more acidic your mouth is, the more likely these viruses will thrive. Certain irritants can cause them to erupt, and some people get them after overexposure to the sun. "Fever blisters," as they are sometimes called, can come at the onset of illness such as a cold. Stress can also bring them out -- basically, any of the above causes that will lower your body's resistance. The sore, like a cold virus, generally lasts for 7-10 days. Brushing and/or rinsing with baking soda can help prevent as well as treat, since the basic pH helps counteract the acidity in your mouth. Your dental professional can recommend over-the-counter treatments. And lysine supplements can help with prevention.

"In you I trust. Cause me to know the way that I should walk..."

PSALM 143

I have a friend who says he never gets cavities and he hasn't been to the dentist in years...

It's true that some people inherit very strong enamel that helps prevent cavities, while others unfortunately inherit weaker, thinner enamel on their teeth and are more prone to decay. Diet also plays a part in this scenario, as people who eat a lot of sugary or acidic foods and drinks can get cavities more easily.

But most people who have less tendency for cavities can have a greater tendency for gum disease, especially if they form tartar. In addition, if you rarely see a dental professional, this can compound the problem. We also know, according to research, that historically, people tend to lose more teeth from the effects of gum disease (periodontal disease) than from cavities. So it's a very good idea to see a dental professional to make sure your mouth is healthy.

"How much better is wisdom than gold, and understanding than silver."

PROVERBS 16:16

I am in my early 20s and my parents are not paying for my dentistry anymore. I'm not having any problems with my teeth, so I don't think I need or can afford to see a dentist regularly.

One of the most dangerous ages in our lives is what one might call "the invincible age." When we are used to our parents taking us to the dentist regularly, we sometimes forget how important it is to keep going regularly, and tend to take it for granted. Cavities and gum disease can grow very slowly without showing any symptoms like pain. Eventually what can happen, though, is the "worst-case scenario," where you wake up one night with excruciating pain in your mouth! Quite often, this will occur when the wisdom teeth (third molars) are beginning to erupt, which commonly happens in your late teens or early 20s. Remember that the cleaning and exam portion of dentistry is the least expensive part. And doing this can help prevent a lot of future big expense, pain, and even tooth loss, not to mention other health problems in your body that can be related to mouth infection.

"The wise man looks ahead.
The fool attempts to fool himself and won't face facts."

PROVERBS 14:8

Is it impolite to ask my dentist or hygienist how much my treatment will cost? I am on a very tight budget so I need to know.

The best person to ask in the dental office is the person who handles the insurance and financial arrangements. But you might want to ask the dentist or hygienist if there are any less expensive alternative treatments for you.

Sometimes people will put off expensive work, but it's best not to do this if you can help it, because often damage or decay to your teeth can get worse, which can cause pain and even more costly treatment.

"So do not throw away your confidence; it will be richly rewarded. You need to persevere..."

HEBREWS 10:35-36

My dentist is recommending some treatment for me: He has advised me that I have some cavities. But I think I'll wait awhile and put aside some extra money for this. I know my insurance won't cover the whole cost.

Most dental offices have various payment options, and it's not really wise to put off treatment if you have cavities, because the cavities will, of course, get larger. And often, as a result, this will require even more expensive treatment, not to mention the possibility of pain as the decay grows closer to the nerves in the tooth.

Remember, too, that as the end of the year approaches you will be losing whatever dental benefits you have for that year, as they do not carry over. Try to take advantage of your benefits. Your dental office financial contact can help you decide what payment options are best for you.

"For then you will make your way prosperous,
and then you will have good success...do not be afraid.. .""

JOSHUA 1:8-9

I started going to the dentist very late in life. I don't remember, as a young child, going to the dentist very much. I just became a regular dental patient as an adult and understood its importance.

As I get older now, I am wondering whether I will be able to keep my teeth forever.

In the "olden days," people didn't go to the dentist unless they had an emergency and quite often were in pain. And in many other countries across the world, this is still true. But here in the United States, dentistry has become more and more preventive. True, it is said that only about 60 percent of the population in this country go to the dentist, and of that number, a smaller percentage choose to undergo regular preventive dentistry. However, gone are the days when we expected to lose all our teeth, because with a few simple routine visits like dental cleanings and exams, most people can keep their teeth for their entire lifetime. It's never too late to start taking care of your teeth!

"Receive my instruction, and not silver, and knowledge rather than choice gold; for wisdom is better than rubies..."

PROVERBS 8:10-11

I plan on just getting dentures someday.
I can't afford to go to the dentist!

This idea used to be more common 100 years ago, and still is common in many countries outside of the United States. But dentistry has changed so much since then that we now know there are other, better alternatives. First of all, if you go to the dentist regularly, it's not necessarily that expensive; prevention is the key. Waiting to go to the dentist until you have a problem can be very costly. True, some people, because of accidents or illness, might need to get full dentures. But think about this: Having dentures can give you a whole new set of challenges. And infection in your mouth that continues for a long time, while you wait for your teeth to deteriorate, can affect your whole body's health. In addition, over time, as your gum tissue naturally shrinks, even if you have dentures, denture relines are necessary, to make sure you have a good fit. Otherwise, your dentures can be uncomfortable, and it can be difficult to chew and eat, making this another possible problem. Then, you might tend to resort to softer foods that may not be as good as the fibrous foods you need for digestion.

With a few easy measures, such as getting your teeth cleaned and checked regularly, the average person can keep his/her teeth for a lifetime. Appreciate what your teeth do for you; don't take them for granted. Your smile, the ability to eat all the foods helping your digestion, and your general health and well-being are all very important. Gone are the days when we all expected to eventually lose our teeth...it's a new day!

"God wants us to have life and have it more abundantly."

JOHN 10:10

I have a big space between my teeth where the food always collects. Can't the dentist just fill up the space?

Almost everyone has at least one area in the mouth that is an irritating food trap. There can be many reasons for this problem. First, our gums tend to recede naturally as we get older, causing more space overall. Possibly, the problem can be an ill-fitting crown or even a loose or lost filling. This can often be corrected by the dentist. Another cause might be a symptom of periodontal (gum) disease. Consulting a dentist or hygienist can help with this problem, and sometimes referral to a periodontist (gum specialist) is needed. Periodontists can actually perform laser treatments to rebuild the bone, and tissue grafting can, if necessary, help fill the space.

The best solution for home care is to use interproximal dental items such as a brush, pick, or water irrigator, to help keep the gum healthy and prevent gum tissue from receding even more, causing an even bigger space.

"The intelligent man is always open to new ideas. In fact, he looks for them."

PROVERBS 18:15

I just had a new filling done at my dental office and my tooth is still sensitive...

There can be several reasons why a tooth is still be sensitive after treatment. If the filling is large and close to your tooth's nerve, it can be sensitive longer. Cold sensitivity and sensitivity to touch are common and normally go away over time; this can take a month or more. A crack in a tooth can cause sensitivity, too. Any place where your root is newly exposed (which happens as a reaction to a filling near the gum, as your gum can pull away a bit) can cause sensitivity. This is because your root is not covered by enamel, so the nerves are closer to the surface. Sometimes you might need to have your dentist check your bite: As can happen, a new filling might have a high spot that needs to be adjusted. But if the sensitivity is getting worse -- especially if your tooth is sensitive to hot -- it's best to seek professional advice, if you are concerned, at your dental office.

"Do not be anxious about anything, but in every situation, by prayer and petition, with thanksgiving, present your requests to God."

PHILIPPIANS 4:6

My dentist is advising me to get a crown on one of my teeth

Crowns ("caps") are a great solution for a tooth damaged either from decay or from cracking/chipping, or when a tooth has so much filling in it that the natural structure of the tooth has been lost. There are many different types of crowns. Porcelain crowns look the most natural, but this type of crown is less strong than a gold crown. Gold is a good choice for a tooth in the back of your mouth for obvious aesthetic reasons, and it is also the strongest. Another type of crown is a ceramic crown. Stainless steel is very inexpensive but not very aesthetically pleasing; it is often used with small children, who have baby teeth that will soon be replaced with their permanent teeth.

It's important to remember that crowns sometimes need to be replaced, because as our gum tissue recedes naturally over time, the root surface is exposed. Roots of the teeth aren't covered by enamel, so their structure is not as decay-resistant.

A veneer, different from a full crown, is a nice aesthetic choice for front teeth. It can be described as similar to an acrylic nail for fingernails. There are also onlays and inlays that are a good option over amalgams ("silver fillings"). Onlays/inlays can also be made of various materials like gold or porcelain. Fillings can also be tooth-colored. Your dentist will determine what treatment is best for you.

"Friendly suggestions are as pleasant as perfume."

PROVERBS 27:9

I just got a new crown (cap) and was surprised that my dental insurance didn't cover more of the cost...

All dental insurance plans have different coverage amounts -- some companies offer better coverage than others. Understand, though, that if you have $1,000 per year coverage, for example, you cannot use the entire amount for a crown. Different amounts are portioned for different treatments, and there may be a co-pay amount you are responsible for. In addition, there can be a waiting period for coverage of a crown being redone on the same tooth, or if you have recently signed up for the insurance coverage.

The best thing to do is to contact your insurance company directly, before you have your treatment, so you understand exactly what amount will be covered. And be thankful for whatever coverage you have: Some people don't have any dental insurance at all...

"Always pursue what is good both for yourselves and for all."

1 THESSALONIANS 5:15

I have a space in my mouth where I lost a tooth, and my dentist is recommending an implant...

Dental implants are very popular now, and many people have them. They have actually been around for more than 40 years, and even though a partial denture is another option, for just a little additional cost, implants can last a lifetime. Titanium is the product normally used for the post that is placed in the bone and a crown is then attached to this. Sometimes, a periodontist or oral surgeon can even do a special procedure to increase your bone support if necessary. Of course, once the implant is placed, it will require special cleaning devices for you to use at home. There are many good products available, such as a water irrigator. You will want to consult a dental professional to determine whether you are a good candidate for this option. But it's also most important to try to avoid losing teeth, as this can create a "domino effect." A space can cause your other teeth to shift, possibly causing jaw pain and tooth wear, chipping and cracking. This can happen, as you are overusing the neighboring teeth and your bite is off.

"...In quietness and confidence shall be your strength."

ISAIAH 30:15

My parents are getting older and I am concerned about their dental health...

There are many changes that occur in our bodies as we get older. Our taste buds can change, and that affects a person's appetite and eating habits. Food may no longer taste as good in general, but our taste buds for sweets are still going strong! So, there can be a tendency to prefer sweets; this can create a condition called "adult onset decay." Fluoride rinses can help with this problem. Our gums naturally tend to recede as well, causing spaces or food traps between our teeth. Interdental brushes, picks, and water irrigators, along with floss, can help with this. Osteoporosis can also creep up on the elderly, but we know that the jawbone is normally the last area to be affected by it. Periodontal disease can also become a problem, as it becomes more difficult to clean our teeth. Antibacterial rinses can help, as well as more frequent visits to the dentist. Electric toothbrushes can help with dexterity issues.

If a person is unable to get to the office, dentists can often make house calls. In some states where dental hygienists are permitted to legally practice independently, they can also make house calls.

"But I have trusted in Your loving kindness.
My heart will be full of joy because You will save me."

PSALM 13:5

I have a full upper denture and a lower partial denture. Do I still need to go to the dentist, and what's the best way to clean my dentures?

Even people who have two full dentures need to see a dental professional. And even if you clean your dentures at home, they still can collect plaque, tartar, and stain, plus bacteria. Dentures can be cleaned more thoroughly by a dental professional, and they need to be checked for a possible necessary reline, as your gum tissue continues to recede over time. A general oral exam should also be done regularly to check for inflammation, infection, or possible lesions.

The best way to clean your dentures at home is to soak them daily in a tablet made for this, added to water. Afterwards, of course, rinse and brush your dentures thoroughly.

"Cleanliness is next to Godliness."

JOHN WESLEY, 1778

My child just had an accident and lost one of the permanent teeth...

Whether you are a child or an adult, if a tooth is lost before the normal time it can be a big problem, because all the neighboring teeth can then shift position. This can negatively affect your normal occlusion (bite). As the teeth shift, this can ultimately affect your jaw, causing TMJ problems. Also, it can eventually lead to the need for braces (orthodontics). It can make healthy chewing or biting more difficult if not corrected, causing chipping or cracking of the teeth. All of this can affect your nutrition, general health, and chances for a long and happy life, as the "domino effect" takes place.

It's best to get advice from your dental professional when you or your child loses a tooth. If you have the tooth that came out (mainly true for a permanent tooth), you can place it either in the inside crevice of your cheek or in milk; try not to rinse the tooth too much, as you might damage the delicate fibers needed for reattachment. Often, the tooth can be reattached.

"The wise man is known by his common sense, and a pleasant teacher is the best."

PROVERBS 16:21

My child is active in sports and my dental professional is recommending a mouthguard...

Mouthguards have been used in professional sports such as boxing and football for many years. They are also very important for children, as well as adults, who are active in contact sports. So, a mouthguard would be highly recommended to prevent damage to the teeth. Dental offices are able to make these very easily.

"...But those who hope in the Lord will renew their strength.
They will soar on wings like eagles; they will run and
not grow weary; they will walk and not be faint."

ISAIAH 40:30

I am interested in whitening my teeth -- is it safe?

Cosmetic whitening is very popular now, and it is one way to help reverse your teeth's appearance of aging -- after all, I believe one of the first things people notice about you is your face and your smile. Naturally, you want to be confident, when you smile, that your teeth are looking presentable.

There are two categories of whitening: The first, over-the-counter products, can be effective for many people and are less expensive, but the whitening effect is usually about half that of the second option, in-office treatments. One type of in-office treatment can be done by a faster whitening, accomplished with a special light that speeds up the whitening process; one appointment usually lasts a little over an hour. Or, you may choose to have trays made in the dental office for your upper and lower teeth. These fit your teeth for use at home with a whitening gel. Remember that your teeth are living things, so it's important to be careful not to use this product too often -- maybe every six months. You will need to do touch-ups regardless of which treatment you choose, because your teeth tend to revert to their former shade. It's also advisable to limit staining products like coffee or smoking during the at-home process; your teeth are porous and can absorb the stain more than the whitening gel, giving you less effective results.

Some people experience tooth sensitivity with whitening gel, either in their teeth or gum tissue, or both. There is a solution for this: Desensitizing toothpastes can help, and advice from your dental professional is also recommended. Whitening your teeth is, of course, only one part that contributes to your whole person, but it's a fun thing to do if you desire!

"Your beauty should not come from outward adornment...
It should be that of your inner self, the
unfading beauty of a gentle and quiet spirit..."

1 PETER 3:3-4

My dentist has advised me to see an orthodontist -- why do I need this?

It's a good idea to see an orthodontist for a screening, and children are advised to do this around age 7, while the jawbone is still forming. Sometimes people look at their teeth and think, based on their anterior (front) teeth, that aesthetically the teeth look OK -- not too bad or crooked. There are lots of other important factors to be considered, though. If your teeth are crowded, it can become increasingly difficult to keep them clean and healthy. This can eventually lead to gum disease and cavities, and possibly tooth loss. Another factor to consider is your bite (occlusion). If your bite is not correct, it can be difficult to chew, and it can also cause TMJ problems that can be very painful.

Adult orthodontics are very popular now for people who required braces as a child but did not get them. Also, ortho "relapse" can occur even if the person has already had braces. Again, a professional can give you the best advice.

"Listen to advice and accept discipline,
and at the end you will be counted among the wise."

PROVERBS 19:20

I would like to straighten my teeth, but I work with the public in my job, and I would really be self-conscious about how this would look. I wish I had been able to get braces as a child, but now I wonder if it's too late?

Actually, adult orthodontics is one of the biggest trends in dentistry right now. And there is a treatment for straightening your teeth that doesn't involve metal bands or brackets. Clear, tooth-colored bonding material can be used so that not much shows except the wire. Another popular orthodontic treatment is comprised of a series of clear trays that are virtually invisible. There are different trays that fit over your teeth; then, you simply switch them regularly as your teeth-straightening progresses. You should ask a dental professional about these procedures.

"A wise man will hear and grow in learning."

PROVERBS 1:5

I inherited permanent teeth that, unfortunately, aren't so pretty to look at. And over the years it has gotten worse, as my teeth have become less white and also chipped. I've tried cosmetic whitening over-the counter products and it hasn't really helped that much.

Cosmetic dentistry can help, and you do have several options for your front teeth that you should check into. One beautiful choice is veneers, comprised of a thin layer of porcelain similar in description to acrylic nails. The layer is cemented to your tooth and can give your teeth the perfect appearance you desire. Another option would be bonding on your front teeth; this is less expensive, though it may not be as attractive. Caps or crowns can also be created. Your dentist can determine which is the best choice for you. And you can decide how much you are willing to spend, as these options have varying price ranges.

**"...Make your ear open to wisdom.
Turn your heart to understanding."**

PROVERBS 2:2

What if I should have a dental emergency while out-of-town travelling?

Obviously, if you are in pain and are not sure what to do, advice from a pharmacist can help. Some people may choose to go to the emergency room or urgent care facility. Incidentally, it's best to seek a dental professional. If you can get advice from someone you trust, this is helpful. In any case, you might want to check your insurance coverage first. And as a rule, dentists and hygienists are usually very kind to anyone in this situation, going out of their way to treat people with dental emergencies.

"God says, 'Why are you so angry? Why is your face downcast?
If you do what is right will You not be accepted?"

GENESIS 4:6-7

With all the millions of bacteria everywhere, I worry about whether my dental office is clean enough...

There are signs you can look for that can help tell you whether your office is safe for you and your family. One indication can be how clean the reception area is: Outdated magazines and dusty furniture can sometimes be a sign that the office in general is not clean enough. Pay attention to whether the dental workers wash their hands after entering the room, and whether they always wear gloves -- preferably non-latex -- when working in your mouth. A good dental office adheres to OSHA standards by law, requiring that additional items be worn regularly, such as masks and protective eyewear. Ask questions, and your dental hygienist, dentist, and assistants will be happy to answer them. It's very important that you feel comfortable in your office!

"The wise man is glad to be instructed, but a self-sufficient fool falls flat on his face."

PROVERBS 10:8

Our veterinarian is advising us that our pet needs to get its teeth cleaned...

Animals -- that is, cats and dogs primarily -- do form tartar often, just like people. And this can lead to gum infection, bad breath, and eventual tooth loss, as well as other health problems. If your pet will let you brush its teeth, there are toothpastes sold at your vet's office that are specially made for animals; it's not advisable to use human toothpaste on pets, as this will make them sick. There are also tartar control products for sale that help, made specifically for pets. Certain types of "people food" can contribute to tartar buildup, too.

Your veterinarian can answer all your questions and can advise you best on your pet's treatment. The vet can professionally clean pets' teeth in the office.

**"Then God said, 'Let the earth bring into being things after their kind and everything that moves upon the ground'
...And God saw that it was good."**

GENESIS 1:24-25

GLOSSARY
OF DENTAL TERMINOLOGY

Abrasion
Mechanical wear on the tooth, often on the front of the tooth at the gumline. Can often be caused by brushing incorrectly.

Abfraction
Different from abrasion. A notch at the front of the tooth at the gumline. Caused by clenching, grinding, and/or malocclusion.

ADA
American Dental Association. The governing body for dentists.

ADHA
American Dental Hygienists' Association. The governing body for dental hygienists.

Amalgam
An alloy or blend of materials containing mercury. Used for dental fillings.

Anterior teeth
Front teeth, vs. posterior (back) teeth.

Attrition
In dentistry, a wearing down of the bite or chewing surfaces of the teeth.

Bicuspids
Means "two points." The teeth directly behind the cuspids ("canine " or "eye" teeth). Also called premolars.

Bitewings
Dental radiographs (x-rays). Taken usually with the dental exam. The patient bites on the x-ray holder tab. Helps check for interproximal decay of the teeth.

Bruxism
A condition in which a person grinds or clenches the teeth. Often done while sleeping. Can cause abfractions as well as wear on the chewing surface.

Calculus
Tartar. From the Latin meaning "small pebble," a calcium deposit that forms on the teeth.

Caries
Cavities. Decay of the teeth. Usually requires a filling to stop the decay.

Cementum
Material covering the root of the tooth.

Clenching
See Bruxism.

Crown
A tooth-colored cap placed over the tooth to restore its shape, size, and strength.

Cuspid
A one-pointed tooth in the front corners of the mouth. Primarily used for tearing; e.g., meat. Also called "eye teeth" or "canines."

DDS or DMD
A dentist qualified to practice dentistry. Must be licensed

Dental Assistant
Trained to assist the dentist or hygienist. ("DA")

Dental Hygienist
A licensed professional. Must be registered and trained for two to four years. Legally permitted to work in the patient's mouth, cleaning the teeth, and educating the patient, along with various other responsibilities. ("RDH")

Dentin
Material under the enamel of the tooth.

Enamel
Material that covers the surface of the tooth's crown (the visible part of the tooth in the mouth).

Endodontist
Dental specialist undergoing more training than a general dentist. Performs root canals.

Extract
To remove or take out, especially by effort. In dentistry, refers to pulling a tooth.

Gingiva
Clinical term in dentistry for gum tissue. Found in the mouth, it covers the bone from the neck of the tooth.

Gingivitis
Inflammation of the gum tissue. If not treated, can lead to periodontitis.

Implant
Normally a titanium post that takes the place of the tooth root. Surgically positioned into the jawbone beneath the gumline. Allows the dentist to mount a replacement crown, thus filling the space from an extracted tooth.

Incisor
A front upper or lower tooth. Adapted for cutting. There are four in each arch in front.

Inlay
A filling shaped to fit the tooth cavity , then cemented in place.. Can be composed of different materials; e.g., gold or porcelain. Designed to replace a damaged tooth area.

Maxilla
The upper bone that holds the upper teeth. In humans, it also forms part of the nose and eye socket.

Mandible
The lower jawbone. The largest and strongest bone in the face, holding the lower teeth. Also the last bone in the body to be affected by osteoporosis.

Molar
Large flat teeth at the back of the mouth. Used primarily to grind food during chewing.

OSHA (Occupational Safety and Health Administration)
The federal agency charged with enforcement of safety and health legislation in dentistry, as well as medical and other business.

Occlusion
In dentistry, the relationship between the upper and lower teeth that occurs during chewing or at rest.

Onlay
In dentistry, a filling fitted to a prepared tooth cavity, then cemented in place. Usually gold or porcelain. Larger than an inlay, usually covering the entire chewing surface.

Orthodontist
A dental specialist undergoing more training than a general dentist. Trained to straighten the teeth into proper alignment.

Pedodontist
Also known as a pediatric dentist. Specializing in children's dental health and care, normally up to the age of 18 years old.

Periapical
Refers to the area around the apex or tip of a tooth. Can also mean a radiograph to show the tissue around the tooth.

Periodontium
"Perio," in Latin, meaning "around the tooth." "Dontium" refers to the tooth. A periodontist is a dental specialist who treats periodontal disease of the gum tissue and bone surrounding the tooth. Requires more training than a general dentist.

Plaque
A sticky film that coats the teeth and contains bacteria. Also called biofilm.

Prophy / Prophylaxis.
A measure taken to maintain health and prevent the spread of disease. In dentistry, a prophy or dental cleaning is primarily performed by the hygienist.

Prosthodontics
The branch of dentistry that deals with the restoration and maintenance of oral function by the replacement of missing teeth and other oral structures, or by artificial devices or prostheses such as full or partial dentures.

Pulp
The chamber inside the tooth that contains the nerves, blood supply, and connective tissue; what keeps the tooth alive.

Sulcus
The natural gingival space found between the tooth and gum tissue surrounding the tooth. Normally, this space is cleaned with a toothbrush and floss at home and by a hygienist in the dental office

Temporomandibular joint (TMJ)
The joint where the jawbone connects to the temporal bones of the skull in front of the ear. Can refer to TMJ dysfunction causing pain. Causes can include injury, malaligned teeth, etc. Can be treated by a dental professional.

ACKNOWLEDGMENTS

The author wishes to acknowledge all the very knowledgeable dental employers and staff who have provided invaluable information throughout the years. This has helped me to grow wise and proficient, teaching me the value of kindness, perseverance, and dedication to my profession, ultimately making me a much better person.

Thanks especially to Dr. Dana Takashima, who has been so kind as to proofread my work and to give me a fine example of what dentistry should be.

An additional acknowledgement goes to Sherpa Research Centre for their kind contribution of research-related information on page 8 of this publication.

And lastly, a big acknowledgment and thank you to Lauren Granger, a fellow author, and my daughter, Nicole Repasky, as well as my stepson James Mawae, all of whom have stood by me, giving me information and great patience and support. Without them, this book never would have come to fruition....

"For I know the plans I have for you," says the Lord.
"They are plans for good and not disaster,
to give you a future and a hope."

JEREMIAH 29:11

I hope this little book has helped you with good information that you can use. We all want to live long and happy lives. The more information we have, the easier it can be to attain our goal. And we know, of course, that ignorance is NOT bliss.

To be able to smile with confidence is an attainable goal, and a healthy mouth is key to this. A smile also has an amazing effect on our brain chemistry. When we smile, it releases brain chemicals (endorphins), which have a psychological as well as physiological effect on us. And, of course, this has a wonderful effect on others who are lucky enough to see us smiling; our emotions affect us as well as others. So, I wish for much joy for you in your life always!

"A cheerful heart is good medicine."

PROVERBS 17:22